HASHIMOTO DIET RECIPES FOR SENIORS

Easy-to-Prepare Delicious and Nutritious Meals for Optimal Thyroid Health

Smart Desty

TABLE OF CONTENTS

INTRODUCTION

Jane sat in her peaceful cottage tucked away among whispering pines, her fingertips running along the worn edges of a cookbook. Her days had settled into a calm pattern interspersed with the soft beats of existence. Beneath the serene exterior, however, Jane struggled with the effects of Hashimoto's thyroiditis, a disease that had progressively drained her of her vitality and left her feeling lost.

She opened the cookbook one morning, hoping to find nourishment and vigor on its first page as sunlight streamed through the kitchen window. The smell of herbs and healthy ingredients filled the kitchen as she followed the carefully designed recipes for thyroid health. She turned every meal into a ritual and set out on a determined path to wellbeing.

Nutrient-dense foods caused Jane to feel a little differently with every bite. The old sense of heavy exhaustion started to fade and was replaced with a fresh energy. Her afternoons got busier, her evenings more peaceful, and her mornings more colorful. Cooking had become a self-care ritual for her, demonstrating her tenacity and will to live a life full of energy again.

Jane's battle with Hashimoto's took on a new depth as the weeks stretched into months. The cookbook turned into her dependable friend, assisting her on her journey to recovery and wholeness, so she no longer felt alone in her fight. As she perfected each recipe, she learned that food has the ability to boost one's spirit in addition to nourishing the body.

During her introspective periods, Jane was amazed at her own progress. Once foreign, the cookbook's pages now carried the scars of her journey—a trip filled with modest successes and quiet achievements. Not only did she see the sky and trees outside her kitchen window, but she also saw a landscape full of possibilities and promise.

Jane realized that living with Hashimoto's disease required more than merely managing her illness as she sat at her kitchen table with a grin on her face. Instead, she had to learn to embrace life and be resilient. Through the comfort of a basic cookbook and the sustenance it provided, Jane discovered not only health meals but also a recipe for a fulfilling life.

Understanding Hashimoto's Thyroiditis

Hashimoto's thyroiditis is a journey that affects all facets of life, not just a medical disease. Many people receive the diagnosis after experiencing symptoms that are inexplicable for months or even years, including persistent exhaustion, weight gain that seems out of the blue, dry skin, hair loss, and a constant feeling of coldness. It's a difficult and unpredictable path that frequently leaves people impacted looking for clarification and comfort.

An autoimmune disease, such as Hashimoto's thyroiditis, occurs when the body's immune system unintentionally targets its own tissues. This time, it goes after the thyroid gland, a little gland at the base of the neck that resembles a butterfly. The thyroid gland is essential for controlling energy levels, metabolism, and the balance of hormones in the body. Its capacity to create hormones is compromised when it is attacked, resulting in a variety of symptoms that can greatly affect day-to-day functioning.

Taking care of Hashimoto's might be especially difficult for elderly people. Ageing naturally already causes a number of physiological alterations and health issues. It can be daunting to add an autoimmune disease to the mix. Nonetheless, it's critical to keep in mind that symptoms can be controlled and quality of life enhanced with the appropriate strategy. Dietary manipulation is one of the most powerful tools at your disposal to do this.

The Purpose of a Senior Hashimoto Diet

Our dietary requirements change as we become older. Seniors frequently need higher doses of specific nutrients to keep their health and wellbeing. The body's capacity to absorb and make use of these nutrients may also decline at the same time. This emphasizes how important it is for older persons to have a diet high in nutrients, especially if they have an autoimmune disease like Hashimoto's thyroiditis.

The Hashimoto diet is specifically tailored to meet the dietary requirements of individuals with Hashimoto's disease while also reducing inflammation and promoting thyroid function. There are many advantages to this diet for senior citizens. It can aid in the management of symptoms including exhaustion, joint pain, and cognitive decline, all of which can be made worse by unhealthful eating habits. A balanced diet can also enhance general health, increase vitality, and enhance quality of life.

The author of "Hashimoto Diet Recipes for Seniors," has a thorough awareness of the difficulties and requirements faced by this demographic. Its goal is to offer useful, delectable, and simple recipes that promote thyroid health and general wellbeing. More than that, though, it is a traveling companion that gives you support, understanding, and the reassurance that you are not alone in this.

Diet Is Crucial for Managing Hashimoto's

Food serves as medicine in addition to being fuel. A healthy diet can help the body achieve hormonal balance, lessen inflammation, and supply the nutrients it needs to operate at its best. Certain foods have the ability to either worsen or improve symptoms in people with Hashimoto's. The secret to controlling this illness is knowing which meals to eat and which to avoid.

The anti-inflammatory nature of the Hashimoto diet is one of its main tenets. Numerous common meals can exacerbate inflammation, which is a typical trigger for autoimmune flare-ups. By consuming more anti-inflammatory foods, such as fatty fish, leafy greens, nuts, and seeds, you can help lower the frequency and intensity of symptoms as well as soothe your immune system.

Furthermore, the Hashimoto diet frequently highlights how crucial it is to avoid gluten. Some Hashimoto's patients may experience immunological reactions and inflammation when exposed to gluten, a protein present in wheat, barley, and rye. Many people discover that their symptoms significantly improve when they cut gluten out of their diet.

However, it's important to consider what to include as well as what to stay away from. For thyroid health, nutrient-dense meals high in zinc, iodine, selenium, and vitamin D are crucial. These nutrients aid in maintaining a healthy immune system and support thyroid gland function. You can give your body the resources it needs to recover and flourish by including a range of these foods in your regular meals.

Adopting a Novel Eating Practice

It might be intimidating to change your diet, particularly if you have loved a certain dish or flavor for many years. Giving up comfort foods you know and love could seem like a big deal. Accepting a new eating style does not, however, require sacrificing flavor or satisfaction. Actually, it can lead to an abundance of delectable and healthful options that will satisfy your palate and nourish your body.

"Hashimoto Diet Recipes for Seniors" is brimming with delectable and cozy foods in addition to being beneficial. These recipes are meant to be simple to make with readily available and reasonably priced components. There are many options to fit your needs and preferences, regardless of your level of cooking expertise or preference for straightforward meals.

As you try these dishes, you'll see that eating well can be satisfying and fun. You'll discover how to prepare meals that promote your health and wellbeing, meals you can enjoy with loved ones, and meals that serve as a reminder that food is a joyful and nourishing food source.

Hashimoto's thyroiditis management is a journey that calls for tolerance, perseverance, and an openness to trying new things. The key is figuring out what suits your body and way of life the best. This book is meant to be your constant companion, giving you the information, motivation, and resources you require to transform your life for the better.

Recall that you are not by yourself. Hashimoto's disease affects millions of people worldwide, but they manage their symptoms and lead active, satisfying lives. You are making a significant progress in your quest for greater health by taking charge of your food. You are giving yourself the power to feel better, be more energetic, and fully enjoy life.

Treat yourself with kindness as you set out on this trip. It's acceptable to go cautiously at first because change takes time. No matter how tiny, acknowledge your accomplishments and don't let losses depress you. You have the chance to promote your health and nourish your body with every meal.

Here is where you may get "Hashimoto Diet Recipes for Seniors." As you take control of your health and wellbeing, may this book serve as a source of inspiration, solace, and direction. One delectable meal at a time, we can together walk the route to greater health.

CHAPTER 1: GETTING STARTED

The Hashimoto Diet's Fundamentals

It is crucial to have a firm grasp of the fundamentals before starting any new nutritional endeavor. For patients with Hashimoto's thyroiditis, an autoimmune disease in which the immune system targets the thyroid gland, the Hashimoto diet is intended to help control symptoms and enhance general health. Here, we'll dissect the core ideas of the Hashimoto diet, emphasize important nutrients, and offer helpful starting advice.

Fundamental Ideas

1. Anti-inflammatory Foods: For those with Hashimoto's disease, chronic inflammation is a major problem. Foods high in antioxidants can help lower inflammation and improve general health. Prioritize eating a range of fruits and vegetables, lean meats, and good fats. Leafy greens, berries, nuts, seeds, and fatty fish like salmon are a few excellent choices.

2. Gluten-Free: Reducing gluten in the diet has been shown to assist many Hashimoto's sufferers have fewer symptoms. A protein included in wheat, barley, and rye called gluten may cause an immunological reaction in certain individuals. Choose gluten-free grains such as rice, quinoa, and oats.

3. Sugar Reduction: Sugars that have been refined might aggravate inflammation and cause other health problems. Cutting back on sugar-filled meals and drinks can aid with symptom management. Alternatively, use natural sweeteners sparingly, such as honey or maple syrup.

4. Foods High in Nutrients: To maintain thyroid function and general health, your body requires a variety of vitamins and minerals. Make sure to incorporate foods high in omega-3 fatty acids, zinc, iodine, vitamin D, and selenium in your diet. These nutrients are essential for immunological and thyroid functioning.

5. Avoiding Goitrogens: Substances known to interfere with thyroid function are known as goitrogens. Goitrogenic foods don't have to be completely avoided, although it's a good idea to restrict their raw forms. Brussels sprouts, cauliflower, and other cruciferous vegetables are common goitrogens. These veggies' goitrogenic qualities can be lessened by cooking them.

Crucial Elements

Focus on including the following vital nutrients in your diet to support the function of your thyroid and your general wellbeing:

1. Selenium: Selenium is essential for the synthesis of thyroid hormones and for shielding the thyroid gland from

injury. Fish, sunflower seeds, and Brazil nuts are good sources.

2. Zinc: Zinc aids in the metabolism of thyroid hormones and the immunological system. Zinc is present in foods such as lentils, pumpkin seeds, beef, and poultry.

3. Iodine: Iodine is necessary for the synthesis of thyroid hormones. Even though iodine shortage is uncommon, you should nevertheless incorporate foods like fish, seaweed, and iodized salt in your diet.

4. Vitamin D: Promotes thyroid function and aids in immune system regulation. In addition to being naturally obtained from sun exposure, vitamin D can also be found in supplements, fortified dairy products, and fatty fish.

5. Omega-3 Fatty Acids: These fatty acids promote general health and have anti-inflammatory qualities. Add walnuts, chia seeds, flaxseeds, and fatty fish like mackerel and salmon to your diet.

Essentials for the Kitchen

Having a well-stocked pantry and the appropriate culinary gear are vital for making the Hashimoto diet simpler to follow. To get you started, here are a few necessities:

- Cookware - Food processor or blender: Ideal for creating sauces, soups, and smoothies.

- Sharp Knives and Cutting Board: These are necessary tools for chopping up fruits, veggies, and meats.
- Non-stick Baking Sheets and Pans: Beneficial for baking and cooking a range of foods.
- Instant Pot or Slow Cooker: Excellent for making meals quickly.
- Measuring Cups and Spoons: To ensure precise measures of ingredients.
- Pantry Essentials - Gluten-Free Grains: Buckwheat, rice, quinoa, and gluten-free oats.
- Nuts and Seeds: Flaxseeds, chia seeds, walnuts, and almonds.
- Avocado, coconut, and olive oils are healthy oils.
- Dried or Canted Beans: lentils, black beans, and chickpeas.
- Herbs and Spices: cinnamon, clove powder, ginger, and turmeric.
- Frozen Fruits and Vegetables: Easy choices for morning smoothies and fast lunches.

Planning and Preparing Meals

Maintaining the Hashimoto diet requires careful meal planning and preparation. You may make it easier to stick to your dietary objectives by planning your meals ahead of time and preparing the ingredients. This will ensure that you always have healthy options available. The following advice will help you get started:

1. Schedule Your Meals: Set aside some time every week to organize your meals. Pick dishes that suit your lifestyle and take into account your timetable. Based on your meal plan, create a grocery list to make sure you have everything you need.

2. Batch Cooking: Make a lot of food in advance to freeze or refrigerate later. On hectic days when you don't have time to prepare meals from scratch, this is quite useful. Casseroles, stews, and soups are excellent choices for large-scale cooking.

3. Prep items: Give items a thorough cleaning, cutting, and portioning out once a week. To ensure they're ready to use when you need them, keep them in the refrigerator in airtight containers. Meal prep time can be greatly shortened by doing this.

4. Use Leftovers: To reduce waste and save time, use leftovers in your meal plan. Take a whole chicken, for instance, and utilize the leftovers for soups, salads, and sandwiches throughout the week.

5. Simple dishes: Go for easy dishes that don't need intricate ingredients or a lot of time to prepare. The Hashimoto diet is made easier to follow with the help of this book's simple and easy-to-follow recipes.

While beginning a new diet can be a big adjustment, it can also be a really powerful experience if you have the correct resources, advice, and support. Recall that the Hashimoto diet aims to enhance general health and wellbeing in addition to symptom management. Planning your meals and concentrating on nutrient-dense, anti-inflammatory foods will help you take charge of your health and make adjustments that will benefit your body.

You'll find a range of delectable and simple-to-make dishes in the ensuing chapters, tailored especially for older adults with Hashimoto's thyroiditis. With the aid of these recipes, you can easily adopt the Hashimoto diet's tenets into your everyday routine, maintain your nutritional objectives, and reap the rewards of increased vitality and health.

Be kind to yourself when you set out on this trip. Small steps are OK since change takes time. No matter how tiny, acknowledge your accomplishments and don't let losses depress you. You have the chance to promote your health and nourish your body with every meal. Greetings and best wishes for a happy and healthier you on the Hashimoto diet.

CHAPTER 2: RECIPES FOR BREAKFAST

There's good reason why breakfast is frequently referred to as the most significant meal of the day. Having a healthy, well-balanced breakfast can help you feel your best throughout the day by giving you the energy and nourishment you require. This chapter includes 15 delectable, simple-to-make breakfast recipes tailored especially for older adults with Hashimoto's thyroiditis. Every dish comes with comprehensive instructions to help you prepare delicious and nutritious meals.

1. Green Smoothie with Berries

Components:
- One banana
- One cup frozen mixed berries
- One cup fresh spinach
- One-third cup chia seeds
- One cup almond milk without sugar
- One spoonful honey (optional)

Guidelines:
1. Fill a blender with all the ingredients.
2. Process until smooth.
3. Transfer to a glass and start sipping right away.

Nutritional Details: - 250 calories - 5g of protein and 8g of fat - 42g of carbohydrates - 10g of fiber

2. Breakfast Bowl of Quinoa with Nuts and Berries

Components:

- One cup of cooked quinoa, half a cup of fresh blueberries, and half a cup of sliced fresh strawberries
- 1/4 cup of walnuts, chopped
- Half a teaspoon of ground cinnamon
- One tablespoon of honey
- One cup of almond milk without sugar

Guidelines:

1. Put the cooked quinoa, walnuts, strawberries, and blueberries in a bowl.
2. Sprinkle cinnamon over top and drizzle with honey.
3. Drizzle the mixture with almond milk and mix thoroughly.
4. Present right away.

Nutritional Details:

- 350 calories
- 10g of protein and 15g of fat
- 50g of carbohydrates
- 8g of fiber

3. Spinach and Mushroom Veggie Omelet

Components:

- Two sizable eggs
- 1/4 cup chopped fresh spinach
- 1/4 cup sliced mushrooms
- One tablespoon of olive oil
- To taste, add salt and pepper.

Guidelines:

1. Beat the eggs thoroughly in a small bowl.
2. In a nonstick skillet, warm the olive oil over medium heat.
3. Add the mushrooms and simmer for about 3 minutes, or until softened.
4. Add the spinach and simmer for one minute, or until wilted.
5. Cover the veggies with eggs and cook for 3–4 minutes, or until set.
6. Immediately serve the omelet by folding it in half.

Nutritional Details:

- 220 calories
- 14g of protein - 18g of fat
- 3g of carbohydrates
- 1g of fiber

4. Avocado and Sweet Potato Bowl

Components:
- Half an avocado, sliced
- One medium sweet potato, peeled and cubed
- One tablespoon olive oil
- One tablespoon chopped fresh cilantro
- Half a teaspoon powdered cumin
- To taste, add salt and pepper.

Guidelines:
1. Set oven temperature to 200°C/400°F.
2. Combine salt, pepper, cumin, and olive oil with the sweet potato cubes.
3. After spreading out on a baking sheet, roast for 20 to 25 minutes, or until soft.
4. Put the avocado slices and the roasted sweet potato in a bowl.
5. Add chopped cilantro as a garnish and serve right away.

Nutritional Details:
- 300 calories
- 3g of protein - 21g of fat
- 26g of carbohydrates
- 10g of fiber

5. Smoked salmon and scrambled eggs

Components:
- Two sizable eggs
- 1/4 cup chopped smoked salmon
- One tablespoon of olive oil
- One tablespoon of finely chopped fresh dill
 - Toppings of salt and pepper

Guidelines:
1. Beat the eggs thoroughly in a small bowl.
2. In a nonstick skillet, warm the olive oil over medium heat.
3. Add the eggs and simmer until they start to set, stirring often.
4. Add the smoked salmon and boil the eggs until they are just set.
5. Add some fresh dill as a garnish and serve right away.

Nutritional Details:
- 250 calories
- 18g of protein;
- 20g of fat
- 1g of carbohydrates
- Fiber: 0 g

6. Parfait of Greek Yogurt with Nuts and Seeds

Components:
- One cup of Greek yogurt
- 1/4 cup gluten-free granola
- One-third cup chia seeds
- One spoonful of flaxseeds
- 1/4 cup of fresh berries, to taste
- One tablespoon honey, if desired

Guidelines:
1. Arrange the Greek yogurt, granola, chia, flax, and berry seeds in a glass or bowl.
2. If desired, drizzle with honey.
3. Present right away.

Nutritional Details:
- 350 calories
- 18g of protein
- 12g of fat
- 42g of carbohydrates
- 10g of fiber

7. Poached egg on avocado toast

Components:
- One slice of gluten-free bread and half of mashed avocado
- One big egg and one tablespoon of white vinegar
- Season with salt and pepper
- Add optional red pepper flakes

Guidelines:
1. Toast the bread till it tastes right.
2. Top the toast with mashed avocado.
3. Add white vinegar to a pot of water and bring it to a gentle simmer.
4. Crack the egg into a little bowl and drop it into the water very carefully.
5. Cook for three to four minutes, or until the yolk is still runny but the white is set.
6. Using a slotted spoon, remove the egg and put it on top of the avocado toast.
7. Add salt, pepper, and, if preferred, red pepper flakes for seasoning.

Nutritional Details:
- 280 calories
- 10g of protein and 20g of fat
- 20g of carbohydrates
- 8g of fiber

8. Berries and Chia Pudding

Components:
- 1/2 cup fresh berries
- 1/4 cup chia seeds
- 1 cup unsweetened almond milk
- 1 tablespoon honey
- 1/2 teaspoon vanilla essence

Guidelines:
1. Place the almond milk, honey, vanilla essence, and chia seeds in a bowl.
2. Give it a good stir to blend.
3. For at least four hours, preferably overnight, cover and refrigerate.
4. Before serving, place some fresh berries on top.

Nutritional Details:
- 250 calories
- 6g of protein
- 12g of fat
- 32g of carbohydrates
- 14g of fiber

9. Kale and Sweet Potato Hash

Components:
- 1/2 small onion, diced
- 1 cup fresh kale
- 1 medium sweet potato, peeled and diced
- 1 tablespoon olive oil
- To taste, add salt and pepper.

Guidelines:
1. In a big skillet over medium heat, warm up the olive oil.
2. Cook the sweet potato in diced form for ten minutes or until it is cooked.
3. Add onion and simmer for about 5 minutes, or until transparent.
4. Add the kale and simmer for 2 to 3 minutes, or until wilted.
5. Add salt and pepper to taste and serve right away.

Nutritional Details:
- 220 calories
- 4g of protein;
- 10g of fat
- 30g of carbohydrates
- 6g of fiber

10. Pancakes with Coconut Flour

Components:
- One-fourth cup coconut flour;
- one-fourth teaspoon baking soda
- One-fourth teaspoon salt
- three big eggs
- 1/4 cup almond milk without sugar,
- 1 tablespoon honey,
- 1 teaspoon vanilla essence
- Cooking using coconut oil

Guidelines:
1. Combine the baking soda, salt, and coconut flour in a bowl.
2. Combine eggs, almond milk, honey, and vanilla extract in a separate bowl.
3. Gently stir the dry and wet ingredients together until smooth.
4. In a skillet over medium heat, warm the coconut oil.
5. For every pancake, add 1/4 cup of batter to the skillet.
6. Cook until surface bubbles appear, then turn and continue cooking until golden brown.
7. Garnish with your preferred garnishes.

Nutritional Details:
- 250 calories
- 10g of protein and 18g of fat
- 14g of carbohydrates

- 5g of fiber

11. Blueberries with Baked Oatmeal

Components:
- Two cups of rolled oats free of gluten and one teaspoon of baking powder
- One-half teaspoon of cinnamon
- 1/4 tsp salt
- 1/4 cup honey
- 2 cups almond milk without added sugar
- One big egg, one tsp vanilla extract, and one cup of fresh blueberries

Guidelines:
1. Set oven temperature to 175°C/350°F.
2. Mix the oats, cinnamon, baking powder, and salt in a big bowl.
3. Combine the honey, almond milk, egg, and vanilla essence in a separate bowl.
4. Pour thoroughly combine the wet and dry components.
5. Add the blueberries and fold.
6. Transfer mixture to baking dish that has been oiled.
7. Bake for 35 to 40 minutes, or until the oatmeal is set and the top is golden.
8. Present warm.

Nutritional Details:
- 250 calories
- 6g of protein and 7g of fat

- 42g of carbohydrates
- 6g of fiber

12. Bowl of green smoothie

Components:
- One frozen banana
- One half avocado
- One cup of raw spinach
- Half a cup of almond milk without sugar
- One-third cup chia seeds
- One tablespoon honey, if desired
- Topped with coconut flakes, granola, and fresh berries

Guidelines:
1. In blender, combine frozen banana, avocado, spinach, chia seeds, almond milk, and honey.
2. Process until smooth.
3. Transfer to a bowl and garnish with coconut flakes, granola, and fresh berries.
4. Present right away.

Nutritional Details:
- 300 calories
- 6g of protein
- 18g of fat
- 34g of carbohydrates
- 12g of fiber

13. Banana Toast with Almond Butter

Components:
- One slice of bread without gluten
- Two tablespoons of almond butter
- One sliced banana
- One tsp of chia seeds
- One teaspoon honey, if desired

Guidelines:
1. Toast the bread till it tastes right.
2. Apply toast with almond butter.
3. Place slices of banana on top.
4. Top with chia seeds and, if desired, honey drizzle.
5. Present right away.

Nutritional Details:
- 320 calories
- 8g of protein
- 18g of fat
- 34g of carbohydrates
- 7g of fiber

14. Eggs and avocado in a breakfast salad

Components:
- Two sizable eggs
- Double-cup mixed greens
- 1/4 cup of halved cherry tomatoes
- 1/2 sliced avocado
- One tablespoon each of lemon juice and olive oil
- To taste, add salt and pepper.

Guidelines:
1. Boil for 8 to 10 minutes, then let eggs cool before peeling.
2. Put the cherry tomatoes, avocado, and mixed greens in a bowl.
3. Combine the olive oil, lemon juice, salt, and pepper in a small bowl.
4. Pour the salad with the dressing and toss to mix.
5. Add the sliced eggs to the salad.
6. Present right away.

Nutritional Details:
- 320 calories
- 12g of protein
- 28g of fat
- 10g of carbohydrates
- 6g of fiber

15. Spiced Pumpkin Smoothie

Components:
- Half a cup of canned pumpkin puree
- One frozen banana
- One tablespoon chia seeds
- Half a teaspoon of pumpkin pie spice
- One cup of almond milk without sugar
- One tablespoon honey, if desired

Guidelines:
1. Fill a blender with all the ingredients.
2. Process until smooth.
3. Transfer to a glass and start sipping right away.

Nutritional Details:
- 250 calories
- 4g of protein; 8g of fat
- 42g of carbohydrates
- 10g of fiber

These breakfast recipes are intended to give you the nutrition you need to maintain the health of your thyroid and your general wellbeing. All of the recipes are simple to make and contain components that are helpful in the management of thyroiditis caused by Hashimoto's. Enjoy these tasty and nourishing selections as you start your day!

CHAPTER 3: LUNCH RECIPES

Lunch is a crucial meal for maintaining energy and focus throughout the day, especially for those managing Hashimoto's thyroiditis. A balanced, nutrient-dense lunch can help sustain energy levels and support overall health. In this chapter, we present 15 delicious and easy-to-prepare lunch recipes that align with the principles of the Hashimoto diet. Each recipe includes detailed information to guide you in creating wholesome and satisfying meals.

1. Quinoa and Chickpea Salad

Ingredients:
- 1 cup cooked quinoa
- 1 cup canned chickpeas, drained and rinsed
- 1/2 cup cherry tomatoes, halved
- 1/4 cup cucumber, diced
- 1/4 cup red onion, finely chopped
- 2 tablespoons olive oil
- 1 tablespoon lemon juice
- 1 tablespoon chopped fresh parsley
- Salt and pepper to taste

Instructions:
1. In a large bowl, combine quinoa, chickpeas, cherry tomatoes, cucumber, and red onion.
2. In a small bowl, whisk together olive oil, lemon juice, parsley, salt, and pepper.

3. Pour the dressing over the salad and toss to combine.
4. Serve immediately or refrigerate for up to 2 days.

Nutritional Information:
- Calories: 350
- Protein: 12g
- Fat: 14g
- Carbohydrates: 46g
- Fiber: 9g

2. Turkey and Avocado Lettuce Wraps

Ingredients:
- 8 large lettuce leaves (romaine or butter lettuce)
- 1 cup cooked turkey breast, sliced
- 1 avocado, sliced
- 1/2 cup shredded carrots
- 1/4 cup red bell pepper, sliced
- 2 tablespoons hummus
- Salt and pepper to taste

Instructions:
1. Lay out the lettuce leaves on a clean surface.
2. Spread a small amount of hummus on each leaf.
3. Top with turkey slices, avocado, shredded carrots, and red bell pepper.
4. Season with salt and pepper.
5. Roll up the lettuce leaves and secure with a toothpick if necessary.
6. Serve immediately.

Nutritional Information:
- Calories: 250
- Protein: 20g
- Fat: 16g
- Carbohydrates: 12g
- Fiber: 8g

3. Salmon and Asparagus Salad

Ingredients:

- 4 oz cooked salmon, flaked
- 1 cup fresh asparagus, blanched and chopped
- 2 cups mixed greens
- 1/4 cup cherry tomatoes, halved
- 2 tablespoons olive oil
- 1 tablespoon balsamic vinegar
- Salt and pepper to taste

Instructions:

1. In a large bowl, combine mixed greens, asparagus, and cherry tomatoes.
2. Add the flaked salmon on top.
3. In a small bowl, whisk together olive oil, balsamic vinegar, salt, and pepper.
4. Drizzle the dressing over the salad and toss to combine.
5. Serve immediately.

Nutritional Information:

- Calories: 350
- Protein: 22g
- Fat: 24g
- Carbohydrates: 10g
- Fiber: 5g

4. Lentil Soup with Spinach

Ingredients:
- 1 cup dried lentils, rinsed
- 1 small onion, chopped
- 2 cloves garlic, minced
- 2 carrots, chopped
- 2 celery stalks, chopped
- 1 can (14.5 oz) diced tomatoes
- 4 cups vegetable broth
- 2 cups fresh spinach, chopped
- 1 tablespoon olive oil
- 1 teaspoon ground cumin
- 1 teaspoon paprika
- Salt and pepper to taste

Instructions:
1. In a large pot, heat olive oil over medium heat.
2. Add onion, garlic, carrots, and celery, and cook until softened, about 5 minutes.
3. Add lentils, diced tomatoes, vegetable broth, cumin, paprika, salt, and pepper.
4. Bring to a boil, then reduce heat and simmer for 25-30 minutes, until lentils are tender.
5. Stir in chopped spinach and cook for an additional 5 minutes.
6. Serve hot.

Nutritional Information:- Calories: 280 - Protein: 14g - Fat: 5g - Carbohydrates: 44g - Fiber: 16g

5. Zucchini Noodles with Pesto and Cherry Tomatoes

Ingredients:
- 2 medium zucchinis, spiralized
- 1/2 cup cherry tomatoes, halved
- 1/4 cup pesto sauce (store-bought or homemade)
- 1 tablespoon olive oil
- Salt and pepper to taste

Instructions:
1. Heat olive oil in a large skillet over medium heat.
2. Add zucchini noodles and cook for 2-3 minutes, until slightly tender.
3. Add cherry tomatoes and cook for an additional 1-2 minutes.
4. Remove from heat and toss with pesto sauce.
5. Season with salt and pepper and serve immediately.

Nutritional Information:
- Calories: 200
- Protein: 4g
- Fat: 16g
- Carbohydrates: 14g
- Fiber: 4g

6. Chicken and Avocado Salad

Ingredients:
- 2 cups cooked chicken breast, chopped
- 1 avocado, diced
- 1/2 cup cherry tomatoes, halved
- 1/4 cup red onion, finely chopped
- 2 tablespoons fresh lime juice
- 2 tablespoons olive oil
- 1 tablespoon chopped fresh cilantro
- Salt and pepper to taste

Instructions:
1. In a large bowl, combine chicken, avocado, cherry tomatoes, and red onion.
2. In a small bowl, whisk together lime juice, olive oil, cilantro, salt, and pepper.
3. Pour the dressing over the salad and toss to combine.
4. Serve immediately or refrigerate for up to 1 day.

Nutritional Information:
- Calories: 350
- Protein: 28g
- Fat: 24g
- Carbohydrates: 10g
- Fiber: 6g

7. Quinoa Stuffed Bell Peppers

Ingredients:

- 4 large bell peppers, tops removed and seeded
- 1 cup cooked quinoa
- 1 cup black beans, drained and rinsed
- 1/2 cup corn kernels
- 1/2 cup diced tomatoes
- 1/4 cup chopped red onion
- 1/4 cup chopped fresh cilantro
- 1 teaspoon ground cumin
- 1 teaspoon paprika
- Salt and pepper to taste
- 1/2 cup shredded cheese (optional)

Instructions:

1. Preheat oven to 375°F (190°C).
2. In a large bowl, combine quinoa, black beans, corn, tomatoes, red onion, cilantro, cumin, paprika, salt, and pepper.
3. Stuff each bell pepper with the quinoa mixture.
4. Place stuffed peppers in a baking dish and cover with foil.
5. Bake for 30 minutes, then remove foil and sprinkle with cheese if using.
6. Bake for an additional 10 minutes, until peppers are tender and cheese is melted.
7. Serve hot.

Nutritional Information:- Calories: 300 - Protein: 10g - Fat: 8g - Carbohydrates: 48g - Fiber: 12g

8. Tuna Salad with Olive Oil and Lemon

Ingredients:
- 1 can (5 oz) tuna packed in water, drained
- 1/4 cup chopped celery
- 1/4 cup chopped red onion
- 1/4 cup chopped fresh parsley
- 2 tablespoons olive oil
- 1 tablespoon fresh lemon juice
- Salt and pepper to taste

Instructions:
1. In a bowl, combine tuna, celery, red onion, and parsley.
2. In a small bowl, whisk together olive oil, lemon juice, salt, and pepper.
3. Pour the dressing over the tuna mixture and toss to combine.
4. Serve immediately or refrigerate for up to 2 days.

Nutritional Information:
- Calories: 250
- Protein: 20g
- Fat: 16g
- Carbohydrates: 6g
- Fiber: 2g

9. Spinach and Feta Stuffed Chicken Breast

Ingredients:
- 2 large chicken breasts
- 1 cup fresh spinach, chopped
- 1/4 cup feta cheese, crumbled
- 1 tablespoon olive oil
- 1 teaspoon dried oregano
- Salt and pepper to taste

Instructions:
1. Preheat oven to 375°F (190°C).
2. In a bowl, combine spinach and feta cheese.
3. Cut a pocket into each chicken breast and stuff with the spinach mixture.
4. Secure with toothpicks if necessary.
5. Season the chicken breasts with olive oil, oregano, salt, and pepper.
6. Place chicken in a baking dish and bake for 25-30 minutes, until the chicken is cooked through.
7. Serve hot.

Nutritional Information:
- Calories: 350
- Protein: 40g
- Fat: 18g
- Carbohydrates: 2g
- Fiber: 1g

10. Cauliflower Rice Stir-Fry

Ingredients:
- 1 head cauliflower, grated into rice-sized pieces
- 1 cup mixed vegetables (carrots, peas, bell peppers)
- 2 cloves garlic, minced
- 2 tablespoons soy sauce (gluten-free)
- 1 tablespoon olive oil
- 1 teaspoon sesame oil
- 2 large eggs, beaten
- Salt and pepper to taste

Instructions:
1. Heat olive oil in a large skillet over medium heat.
2. Add garlic and cook for 1 minute, until fragrant.
3. Add mixed vegetables and cook until tender, about 5 minutes.
4. Push the vegetables to the side of the skillet and pour the beaten eggs into the empty space.
5. Scramble the eggs until fully cooked, then mix with the vegetables.
6. Add cauliflower rice, soy sauce, sesame oil, salt, and pepper.
7. Cook for an additional 5 minutes, until cauliflower is tender.
8. Serve hot.

Nutritional Information:
- Calories: 200
- Protein: 10g
- Fat: 12g
- Carbohydrates: 18g
- Fiber: 5g

11. Mediterranean Chickpea Salad

Ingredients:
- 1 can (15 oz) chickpeas, drained and rinsed
- 1/2 cup cherry tomatoes, halved
- 1/2 cup cucumber, diced
- 1/4 cup red onion, finely chopped
- 1/4 cup Kalamata olives, pitted and sliced
- 2 tablespoons olive oil
- 1 tablespoon red wine vinegar
- 1 tablespoon chopped fresh parsley
- Salt and pepper to taste

Instructions:
1. In a large bowl, combine chickpeas, cherry tomatoes, cucumber, red onion, and Kalamata olives.
2. In a small bowl, whisk together olive oil, red wine vinegar, parsley, salt, and pepper.
3. Pour the dressing over the salad and toss to combine.
4. Serve immediately or refrigerate for up to 2 days.

Nutritional Information:
- Calories: 300
- Protein: 10g
- Fat: 14g
- Carbohydrates: 36g
- Fiber: 10g

12. Turkey and Veggie Wraps

Ingredients:

- 4 large lettuce leaves (romaine or butter lettuce)
- 1 cup cooked turkey breast, sliced
- 1/2 cup shredded carrots
- 1/4 cup red bell pepper, sliced
- 2 tablespoons hummus
- Salt and pepper to taste

Instructions:

1. Lay out the lettuce leaves on a clean surface.
2. Spread a small amount of hummus on each leaf.
3. Top with turkey slices, shredded carrots, and red bell pepper.
4. Season with salt and pepper.
5. Roll up the lettuce leaves and secure with a toothpick if necessary.
6. Serve immediately.

Nutritional Information:

- Calories: 250
- Protein: 20g
- Fat: 16g
- Carbohydrates: 12g
- Fiber: 8g

13. Sweet Potato and Black Bean Tacos

Ingredients:
- 2 medium sweet potatoes, peeled and diced
- 1 can (15 oz) black beans, drained and rinsed
- 1/2 teaspoon ground cumin
- 1/2 teaspoon chili powder
- 1 tablespoon olive oil
- Salt and pepper to taste
- 8 small corn tortillas
- 1/4 cup chopped fresh cilantro
- 1/4 cup diced red onion
- Lime wedges for serving

Instructions:
1. Preheat oven to 400°F (200°C).
2. Toss diced sweet potatoes with olive oil, cumin, chili powder, salt, and pepper.
3. Spread on a baking sheet and roast for 20-25 minutes, until tender.
4. In a bowl, combine roasted sweet potatoes and black beans.
5. Warm tortillas in a dry skillet or microwave.
6. Fill each tortilla with the sweet potato and black bean mixture.
7. Top with chopped cilantro and diced red onion.
8. Serve with lime wedges.

Nutritional Information:- Calories: 350
- Protein: 10g   - Fat: 8g
- Carbohydrates: 60g
- Fiber: 12g

14. Thai Chicken Salad with Peanut Dressing

Ingredients:
- 2 cups cooked chicken breast, shredded
- 2 cups shredded cabbage
- 1 cup shredded carrots
- 1/2 cup red bell pepper, sliced
- 1/4 cup chopped fresh cilantro
- 1/4 cup chopped peanuts
- 2 tablespoons peanut butter
- 1 tablespoon soy sauce (gluten-free)
- 1 tablespoon lime juice
- 1 tablespoon honey
- 1 teaspoon sesame oil

Instructions:
1. In a large bowl, combine chicken, cabbage, carrots, red bell pepper, cilantro, and peanuts.
2. In a small bowl, whisk together peanut butter, soy sauce, lime juice, honey, and sesame oil until smooth.
3. Pour the dressing over the salad and toss to combine.
4. Serve immediately or refrigerate for up to 1 day.

Nutritional Information:
- Calories: 400
- Protein: 30g
- Fat: 20g
- Carbohydrates: 28g
- Fiber: 8g

15. Shrimp and Avocado Salad

Ingredients:

- 1 cup cooked shrimp, peeled and deveined
- 1 avocado, diced
- 1/2 cup cherry tomatoes, halved
- 1/4 cup red onion, finely chopped
- 2 tablespoons fresh lime juice
- 2 tablespoons olive oil
- 1 tablespoon chopped fresh cilantro
- Salt and pepper to taste

Instructions:

1. In a large bowl, combine shrimp, avocado, cherry tomatoes, and red onion.
2. In a small bowl, whisk together lime juice, olive oil, cilantro, salt, and pepper.
3. Pour the dressing over the salad and toss to combine.
4. Serve immediately or refrigerate for up to 1 day.

Nutritional Information:

- Calories: 350
- Protein: 18g
- Fat: 24g
- Carbohydrates: 14g
- Fiber: 8g

CHAPTER 4: RECIPES FOR DINNER

Dinner is a crucial meal that, particularly for those treating Hashimoto's thyroiditis, can help balance blood sugar levels and promote a good night's sleep. This chapter offers 15 savory and filling dinner recipes that are specifically designed to promote thyroid health. To guarantee a tasty and nourishing supper, every recipe is created to be simple to prepare and comes with comprehensive instructions.

1. Roasted Vegetables and Quinoa with Baked Salmon

Components:
- 4 fillets of salmon, 4-6 ounces each
- One cup of washed quinoa
- Two cups of mixed veggies, such as broccoli, zucchini, and bell peppers
- Two tsp olive oil
- One sliced lemon
- To taste, add salt and pepper.

Guidelines:
1. Turn the oven on to 400°F, or 200°C.
2. Follow the directions on the package to cook the quinoa.
3. Spread out mixed vegetables on a baking sheet after tossing them with olive oil, salt, and pepper.
4. With the skin side down, place the salmon fillets on the baking sheet.

5. Place slivers of lemon over the fish.
6. Bake for 15 to 20 minutes, or until the veggies are soft and the salmon is cooked through.
7. Over cooked quinoa, serve fish and vegetables.

Nutritional Details:
- 400 calories
- 30g of protein
- 18g of fat
- 30g of carbohydrates
- 6g of fiber

2. Stir-fried Turkey with Vegetables

Components:
- One pound of turkey meat
- Two cups of mixed veggies, such as carrots, snap peas, and bell peppers
- Two minced garlic cloves
- 1 tablespoon finely chopped ginger
- Two tablespoons of gluten-free soy sauce
- A tsp of sesame oil
- To taste, add salt and pepper.
- Prepared quinoa or rice for serving

Guidelines:
1. In a large skillet or wok, heat the sesame oil over medium-high heat.
2. Using a spoon, break up the ground turkey and sauté it until it turns brown.
3. After adding the mixed vegetables, ginger, and garlic, simmer for 5 to 7 minutes, or until the vegetables are soft.
4. Add the pepper, salt, and soy sauce.
5. Serve quinoa or cooked rice with stir-fry.

Nutritional Details:
- 380 calories
- 30g of protein
- 20g of fat
- 20g of carbohydrates
- 4g of fiber

3. Bell peppers stuffed with Mediterranean flavor

Components:
- 4 large bell peppers, seeded and stripped of their tips
- A cup of prepared quinoa
- One 15-oz can of washed and drained chickpeas
- Half a cup of cherry tomatoes
- 1/4 cup pitted and sliced Kalamata olives
- 1/4 cup of feta cheese, crumbled
- Two tsp olive oil
- One-third cup red wine vinegar
- One tablespoon of freshly chopped parsley
- To taste, add salt and pepper.

Guidelines:
1. Turn the oven on to 375°F, or 190°C.
2. The cooked quinoa, chickpeas, cherry tomatoes, olives, feta cheese, olive oil, red wine vinegar, parsley, salt, and pepper should all be combined in a big bowl.
3. Stuff the quinoa mixture inside each bell pepper.
4. Cover the filled peppers with foil after placing them in a roasting dish.
5. Bake the peppers for 30 minutes, then take off the foil and continue baking for another 10 minutes, or until they are soft.
6. Warm up the food.

Nutritional Details: - 350 calories   14g of protein
- 16g of fat   - 40g of carbohydrates   - 10g of fiber

4. Quinoa with Vegetable and Chicken Skewers

Components:
- A one-pound chicken breast, cubed
- Two cups of mixed veggies, including zucchini, cherry tomatoes, and bell peppers
- Two tsp olive oil
- Half a cup of lemon juice
- One teaspoon of oregano, dried
- To taste, add salt and pepper.
- Steamed quinoa ready to eat

Guidelines:
1. Set the grill pan or grill to medium-high heat.
2. Chicken cubes, mixed veggies, lemon juice, olive oil, oregano, salt, and pepper should all be combined in a bowl. Toss in the coat.
3. Put veggies and chicken on skewers.
4. Cook the skewers for 10 to 12 minutes, rotating them halfway through, or until the vegetables are soft and the chicken is cooked through.
5. Slide skewers onto warm quinoa.

Nutritional Details:
- 380 calories
- 35g of protein
- 16g of fat
- 25g of carbohydrates
- 4g of fiber

5. Stir-fried Broccoli with Beef

Components:
- One pound of finely sliced beef sirloin
- 3 cups florets of broccoli
- One sliced red bell pepper
- Two minced garlic cloves
- 1 tablespoon finely chopped ginger
- 1/4 cup gluten-free soy sauce
- Two teaspoons of honey
- 1tsp. of sesame oil
- Enough rice cooked to serve

Guidelines:
1. Mix the sesame oil, honey, and soy sauce in a bowl.
2. In a large skillet or wok, heat the sesame oil over medium-high heat.
3. Cook the beef slices for two to three minutes on each side, or until browned. Take out of the skillet and place aside.
4. To the skillet, add the bell pepper, broccoli, ginger, and garlic. Cook vegetables for 5 to 7 minutes, or until they are crisp-tender.
5. Place the steak back in the skillet and cover everything with the soy sauce mixture. Cook, stirring, for two to three minutes, or until thoroughly heated.
6. Put the stir-fry on top of cooked rice.

Nutritional Details: 420 calories, 35g of protein
- 18g of fat   - 30g of carbohydrates   - 4g of fiber

6. Curry with cauliflower and chickpeas

Components:
- One head of chopped cauliflower
- One 15-oz can of washed and drained chickpeas
- One onion, diced finely
- Two minced garlic cloves
- 1 tablespoon finely chopped ginger
- One 14-oz can of chopped tomatoes
- One 14-ounce can of coconut milk
- Two tsp olive oil
- Two tsp curry powder
- To taste, add salt and pepper.
- Prepared quinoa or rice for serving

Guidelines:
1. In a big pot, warm up the olive oil over medium heat.
2. Add the ginger, garlic, and onion. Simmer for 3–4 minutes, or until tender.
3. Add the curry powder and stir until aromatic, about 1 minute.
4. Add the chickpeas, chopped tomatoes with their liquids, coconut milk, and cauliflower florets.
5. Add pepper and salt for seasoning. After bringing to a boil, lower the heat, and simmer the cauliflower for 20 to 25 minutes, or until it is soft.
6. Serve quinoa or cooked rice with curry.

Nutritional Details:- 380 calories   -12g of protein
- 20g of fat   - 40g of carbohydrates   - 12g of fiber

7. Chicken Breast Stuffed with Spinach and Ricotta

Components:

- Four skinless and boneless chicken breasts
- One cup of freshly chopped spinach
– Half a cup of ricotta
- 1/4 cup of mozzarella cheese, shredded
- Two tsp olive oil
- One tsp of Italian spice
- To taste, add salt and pepper.

Guidelines:

1. Turn the oven on to 375°F, or 190°C.
2. Add chopped spinach, mozzarella and ricotta cheeses, olive oil, salt, pepper, and Italian seasoning to a bowl.
3. Make indentations on each chicken breast, then fill them with the spinach mixture.
4. If needed, use toothpicks to secure.
5. Sprinkle salt and pepper on the outside of the chicken breasts.
6. In a skillet that is ovensafe, warm the olive oil over medium-high heat.
7. Sear chicken breasts till golden brown, 3–4 minutes per side.
8. After moving the skillet to the oven, roast it for 20 to 25 minutes, or until the chicken is thoroughly cooked and its juices run clear.
9. Take off the toothpicks prior to serving.

Nutritional Details: - 380 calories; 40g of protein

- 18g of fat   - 8g of carbohydrates   - 2g of fiber

8. Soup with Lentils and Veggies

Components:
- One cup of washed dried green lentils
- One chopped onion
- 2 sliced carrots
- Two sliced celery stalks
- Two minced garlic cloves
- One 14-oz can of chopped tomatoes
– Six cups broth made of vegetables
- One tablespoon of olive oil
- A teaspoon of thyme, dried
- To taste, add salt and pepper.

Guidelines:
1. In a big pot, warm up the olive oil over medium heat.
2. Add the garlic, celery, carrots, and onion. Simmer for 5 to 7 minutes, or until tender.
3. Once aromatic, simmer for one minute after adding the dried thyme.
4. Add the lentils, tomato juices, and diced tomatoes to the vegetable broth.
5. Add pepper and salt for seasoning. Bring about the lentils to a boil, then lower the heat and simmer for 25 to 30 minutes, or until they are soft.
6. Warm up the food.

Nutritional Details: - 320 calories   - 18g of protein

- 6g of fat   - 50g of carbohydrates   - 20g of fiber

9. Brown rice, shrimp, and vegetables stir-fried

Components:
- One pound of peeled and deveined shrimp
- Two cups of mixed veggies, such as broccoli, snap peas, and bell peppers
- Two minced garlic cloves
- 1 tablespoon finely chopped ginger
- Two tablespoons of gluten-free soy sauce
- 1tsp of sesame oil
- Brown rice cooked and ready to serve
- To taste, add salt and pepper.

Guidelines:
1. In a large skillet or wok, heat the sesame oil over medium-high heat.
2. Add shrimp and fry until pink and opaque, 2 to 3 minutes per side. Take out of the skillet and place aside.
3. Ginger, garlic, and mixed veggies should be added to the skillet. Cook vegetables for 5 to 7 minutes, or until they are crisp-tender.
4. Put the shrimp back in the skillet and cover everything with soy sauce. Cook, stirring, for two to three minutes, or until thoroughly heated.
5. Garnish stir-fried food with cooked brown rice.

Nutritional Details: - 350 calories   - 30g of protein

\- 10g of fat   - 40g of carbohydrates   - 6g of fiber

10. Black bean and Quinoa Stuffed Sweet Potatoes

Components:
- Four medium-sized sweet potatoes
- A cup of prepared quinoa
- One can (15 ounces) of rinsed and drained black beans
- Half a cup of kernel corn
- 1/4 cup of freshly chopped cilantro
- One teaspoon of cumin powder
- One tsp of chili powder
- To taste, add salt and pepper.

Guidelines:
1. Turn the oven on to 400°F, or 200°C.
2. Sweet potatoes should be pierced with a fork and put on a baking sheet.
3. Bake until soft, 45 to 60 minutes.
4. Cooked quinoa, black beans, corn kernels, cilantro, cumin, chili powder, salt, and pepper should all be combined in a bowl.
5. Using a fork, cut open the sweet potatoes and fluff the flesh.
6. Fill sweet potatoes with the mixture of quinoa.
7. Warm up the food.

Nutritional Details:
- 380 calories
- 15g of protein

- 4g of fat
- 75g of carbohydrates
- 12g of fiber

11. Curry of Thai Vegetables with Tofu

Components:

- One block (fourteen ounces) of firm tofu, diced
- Two cups of mixed veggies, such as carrots, snap peas, and bell peppers
- One chopped onion
- Two minced garlic cloves
- 1 tablespoon finely chopped ginger
- One 14-ounce can of coconut milk
- Two tablespoons pasted red curry.
- One tablespoon of gluten-free soy sauce
- One tablespoon of olive oil
- Prepared quinoa or rice for serving
- To taste, add salt and pepper.

Guidelines:

1. In a big pot, warm up the olive oil over medium heat.
2. Add the ginger, garlic, and onion. Simmer for 3–4 minutes, or until tender.
3. Add the red curry paste and stir until aromatic, about 1 minute.
4. Cook the mixed vegetables for five minutes, stirring from time to time.
5. Add soy sauce and coconut milk. After bringing to a boil, lower heat, and simmer for ten minutes.
6. Cook the tofu cubes for a further five minutes, or until they are well heated.

7. Serve quinoa or cooked rice with curry.

Nutritional Details: 420 calories, 20g of protein

- Fat (g): 24 - 35g of carbohydrates   - 8g of fiber

12. Chicken with Lemon Garlic and Roasted Brussels Sprouts

Components:

- Four skinless and boneless chicken breasts
- 2 cups halves and trimmings of Brussels sprouts
- Four minced garlic cloves
- Juiced and zest of two lemons
- Two tsp olive oil
- A teaspoon of thyme, dried
- To taste, add salt and pepper.

Guidelines:

1. Turn the oven on to 400°F, or 200°C.
2. Minced garlic, lemon zest, lemon juice, olive oil, dried thyme, salt, and pepper should all be combined in a bowl.
3. Arrange Brussels sprouts and chicken breasts on a baking pan.
4. Toss to ensure uniform coating of the chicken and Brussels sprouts after adding the lemon-garlic combination.
5. Bake for 25 to 30 minutes, or until Brussels sprouts are soft and chicken is cooked through.
6. Warm up the food.

Nutritional Details:

- 380 calories   - 40g of protein   - 16g of fat

- 20g of carbohydrates   - 8g of fiber

66

13. Squash Noodles paired with Turkey Meatballs

Components:

- One large spaghetti squash
- One pound of turkey meat
- 1/4 cup breadcrumbs or almond flour
- One egg
- 1/4 cup of Parmesan cheese, grated
- One tablespoon of seasoning, Italian
- Two cups marinara sauce (homemade or from the supermarket)
- To taste, add salt and pepper.

Guidelines:

1. Turn the oven on to 400°F, or 200°C.
2. Scoop out the seeds after cutting the spaghetti squash in half lengthwise.
3. Squash halves should be placed on a baking pan, cut side down. Bake until soft, about 40 to 45 minutes.
4. Ground turkey, almond flour, egg, Parmesan cheese, Italian seasoning, salt, and pepper should all be combined in a bowl. Blend until thoroughly blended.
5. Form the mixture into meatballs and arrange them on a parchment paper-lined baking sheet.
6. Meatballs should be baked for 20 to 25 minutes, or until done.
7. Using a fork, scrape the spaghetti squash's meat into strands.
8. Serve meatballs and marinara sauce over spaghetti squash.

Nutritional Details: - 380 calories   35g of protein

- 18g of fat   - 30g of carbohydrates   - 8g of fiber

14. Mango Salsa-Blackened Mahi Mahi

Components:
- 4 fillets of mahi mahi, 4-6 oz each
- One tablespoon of olive oil
- One tablespoon of spice for blackening
- One mango, chopped and peeled
- 1/2 diced red bell pepper
- 1/4 cup coarsely chopped red onion
- 1/4 cup of freshly chopped cilantro
- One tablespoon of lime juice
- To taste, add salt and pepper.

Guidelines:
1. To create the salsa, put the diced mango, red onion, red bell pepper, cilantro, lime juice, salt, and pepper in a bowl. Put aside.
2. Mahi mahi fillets should be rubbed with olive oil, then sprinkled with spice for blackening and lightly pressed to cling.
3. A skillet or grill pan should be heated to medium-high heat.
4. Cook mahi mahi fillets for 3–4 minutes on each side, or until the fish is opaque throughout and flakes readily with a fork.
5. Present mahi mahi fillets with mango salsa on top.

Nutritional Details: - 320 calories   - 30g of protein
- 10g of fat   - 25g of carbohydrates   - 4g of fiber

15. Chickpea with Eggplant Tagine

Components:
- One large eggplant that has been cubed
- One 15-oz can of washed and drained chickpeas
- One chopped onion
- Two minced garlic cloves
- 1 tablespoon finely chopped ginger
- One 14-oz can of chopped tomatoes
- 1/4 cup chopped dried apricots
- 1/4 cup of almonds, sliced
- Two tsp olive oil
- One teaspoon of cumin powder
- One teaspoon of ground cinnamon
- To taste, add salt and pepper.
- Couscous cooked and ready to serve

Guidelines:
1. In a big pot, warm up the olive oil over medium heat.
2. Add the ginger, garlic, and onion. Simmer for 3–4 minutes, or until tender.
3. Add cinnamon and ground cumin and stir. Simmer for one minute, or until aromatic.
4. Add the diced tomatoes with their juices, dried apricots, chickpeas, eggplant cubes, salt, and pepper.
5. Once the eggplant is soft, bring to a boil, then lower the heat and simmer for 25 to 30 minutes.
6. Add sliced almonds and stir.
7. On top of cooked couscous, serve tagine.

Nutritional Details: - 380 calories   - 12g of protein
- 18g of fat   - 50g of carbohydrates   - 12g of fiber

CHAPTER 5: SNACKS AND DESSERTS RECIPES

Maintaining energy levels and satisfying cravings between meals is crucial, especially when managing Hashimoto's thyroiditis. This chapter offers 20 delightful and nutritious snack and dessert recipes designed to support thyroid health. Each recipe is crafted to be easy to prepare and includes detailed instructions for a delicious treat that you can enjoy guilt-free.

1. Greek Yogurt with Berries and Almonds

Ingredients:
- 1 cup Greek yogurt
- ½ cup mixed berries (strawberries, blueberries, raspberries)
- 1/4 cup almonds, chopped
- Honey or maple syrup (optional)

Instructions:
1. Spoon Greek yogurt into a serving bowl.
2. Top with mixed berries and chopped almonds.
3. Drizzle with honey or maple syrup if desired.
4. Serve chilled.

Nutritional Information:
- Calories: 250
- Protein: 20g
- Fat: 12g
- Carbohydrates: 18g

- Fiber: 5g

2. Avocado Chocolate Mousse

Ingredients:
- 2 ripe avocados
- 1/4 cup cocoa powder
- 1/4 cup maple syrup or honey
- 1 teaspoon vanilla extract
- Pinch of salt

Instructions:
1. Scoop avocado flesh into a blender or food processor.
2. Add cocoa powder, maple syrup or honey, vanilla extract, and salt.
3. Blend until smooth and creamy.
4. Chill in the refrigerator for at least 30 minutes before serving.

Nutritional Information:
- Calories: 200
- Protein: 3g
- Fat: 14g
- Carbohydrates: 22g
- Fiber: 8g

3. Apple Slices with Almond Butter and Cinnamon

Ingredients:
- 2 apples, cored and sliced
- 1/4 cup almond butter
- 1 teaspoon ground cinnamon

Instructions:
1. Arrange apple slices on a plate.
2. Spread almond butter over apple slices.
3. Sprinkle with ground cinnamon.
4. Serve immediately.

Nutritional Information:
- Calories: 280
- Protein: 6g
- Fat: 16g
- Carbohydrates: 30g
- Fiber: 8g

4. Energy Bites

Ingredients:
- 1 cup rolled oats
- 1/2 cup almond butter
- 1/4 cup honey or maple syrup
- 1/4 cup ground flaxseed
- 1/4 cup dark chocolate chips
- 1 teaspoon vanilla extract

Instructions:

1. In a bowl, combine rolled oats, almond butter, honey or maple syrup, ground flaxseed, dark chocolate chips, and vanilla extract.
2. Mix until well combined.
3. Roll into bite-sized balls using your hands.
4. Refrigerate for at least 30 minutes before serving.

Nutritional Information (per bite):

- Calories: 120
- Protein: 4g
- Fat: 7g
- Carbohydrates: 12g
- Fiber: 2g

5. Hummus and Veggie Platter

Ingredients:

- 1 cup hummus (store-bought or homemade)
- Assorted vegetables (carrot sticks, cucumber slices, bell pepper strips)

Instructions:

1. Arrange hummus in a serving bowl.
2. Arrange assorted vegetables on a platter.
3. Serve vegetables with hummus for dipping.

Nutritional Information:

- Calories: 180
- Protein: 8g
- Fat: 10g
- Carbohydrates: 18g
- Fiber: 6g

6. Quinoa and Kale Salad

Ingredients:
- 1 cup cooked quinoa
- 1 cup kale, finely chopped
- 1/4 cup dried cranberries
- 1/4 cup chopped walnuts
- 2 tablespoons olive oil
- 1 tablespoon balsamic vinegar
- Salt and pepper to taste

Instructions:
1. In a bowl, combine cooked quinoa, chopped kale, dried cranberries, and chopped walnuts.
2. Drizzle with olive oil and balsamic vinegar.
3. Season with salt and pepper.
4. Toss until well combined.
5. Serve chilled or at room temperature.

Nutritional Information:
- Calories: 280
- Protein: 8g
- Fat: 14g
- Carbohydrates: 32g
- Fiber: 6g

7. Chia Seed Pudding

Ingredients:
- 1/4 cup chia seeds
- 1 cup almond milk (or any milk of choice)
- 1 tablespoon honey or maple syrup
- 1/2 teaspoon vanilla extract
- Fresh berries for topping

Instructions:
1. In a bowl, combine chia seeds, almond milk, honey or maple syrup, and vanilla extract.
2. Stir well to combine.
3. Refrigerate for at least 2 hours, or overnight, until mixture thickens and becomes pudding-like.
4. Stir again before serving and top with fresh berries.

Nutritional Information:
- Calories: 180
- Protein: 5g
- Fat: 9g
- Carbohydrates: 20g
- Fiber: 10g

8. Almond and Date Bars

Ingredients:
- 1 cup almonds
- 1 cup pitted dates
- 1/4 cup unsweetened shredded coconut
- 1 tablespoon coconut oil
- Pinch of salt

Instructions:
1. In a food processor, pulse almonds until finely chopped.
2. Add dates, shredded coconut, coconut oil, and salt.
3. Pulse until mixture sticks together.
4. Press mixture into a lined baking dish and refrigerate for 1 hour.
5. Cut into bars before serving.

Nutritional Information (per bar):
- Calories: 150
- Protein: 4g
- Fat: 8g
- Carbohydrates: 18g
- Fiber: 4g

9. Mango Coconut Smoothie

Ingredients:
- 1 cup frozen mango chunks
- 1/2 cup coconut milk
- 1/2 cup Greek yogurt
- 1 tablespoon honey or maple syrup
- 1/4 cup shredded coconut (optional)

Instructions:
1. Combine frozen mango chunks, coconut milk, Greek yogurt, and honey or maple syrup in a blender.
2. Blend until smooth.
3. Pour into glasses and sprinkle with shredded coconut if desired.
4. Serve immediately.

Nutritional Information:
- Calories: 250
- Protein: 8g
- Fat: 12g
- Carbohydrates: 30g
- Fiber: 4g

10. Baked Apples with Cinnamon and Walnuts

Ingredients:
- 4 apples, cored
- 1/4 cup chopped walnuts
- 1 tablespoon honey or maple syrup
- 1 teaspoon ground cinnamon
- Greek yogurt or whipped cream for serving

Instructions:
1. Preheat oven to 375°F (190°C).
2. Place cored apples in a baking dish.
3. In a bowl, combine chopped walnuts, honey or maple syrup, and ground cinnamon.
4. Spoon mixture into the center of each apple.
5. Bake for 25-30 minutes, until apples are tender.
6. Serve baked apples with a dollop of Greek yogurt or whipped cream.

Nutritional Information:
- Calories: 180
- Protein: 3g
- Fat: 6g
- Carbohydrates: 32g
- Fiber: 6g

11. Spinach and Artichoke Dip

Ingredients:
- 1 cup Greek yogurt
- 1 cup cooked spinach, chopped
- 1 cup canned artichoke hearts, drained and chopped
- 1/4 cup grated Parmesan cheese
- 1/4 cup shredded mozzarella cheese
- 1 clove garlic, minced
- Salt and pepper to taste
- Whole grain crackers or vegetable sticks for dipping

Instructions:
1. Preheat oven to 375°F (190°C).
2. In a bowl, combine Greek yogurt, chopped spinach, chopped artichoke hearts, Parmesan cheese, mozzarella cheese, minced garlic, salt, and pepper.
3. Transfer mixture to a baking dish.
4. Bake for 20-25 minutes, until heated through and bubbly.
5. Serve warm with whole grain crackers or vegetable sticks.

Nutritional Information:
- Calories: 220
- Protein: 18g
- Fat: 10g
- Carbohydrates: 16g
- Fiber: 4g

12. Berry Coconut Chia Popsicles

Ingredients:
- 1 cup mixed berries (strawberries, blueberries, raspberries)
- 1 can (14 oz) coconut milk
- 2 tablespoons chia seeds
- 2 tablespoons honey or maple syrup

Instructions:
1. In a blender, combine mixed berries, coconut milk, chia seeds, and honey or maple syrup.
2. Blend until smooth.
3. Pour mixture into popsicle molds.
4. Insert popsicle sticks and freeze for at least 4 hours, or until solid.
5. Remove popsicles from molds and serve.

Nutritional Information (per popsicle):
- Calories: 120
- Protein: 2g
- Fat: 8g
- Carbohydrates: 12g
- Fiber: 3g

13. Cucumber and Hummus Bites

Ingredients:

- 2 cucumbers, sliced into rounds
- 1 cup hummus (store-bought or homemade)
- Cherry tomatoes for garnish

Instructions:

1. Spread hummus onto cucumber slices.
2. Top each slice with a cherry tomato.
3. Serve chilled.

Nutritional Information:

- Calories: 160
- Protein: 6g
- Fat: 8g
- Carbohydrates: 18g
- Fiber: 6g

14. Coconut Almond Granola Bars

Ingredients:

- 2 cups rolled oats
- 1/2 cup almonds, chopped
- 1/2 cup shredded coconut
- 1/4 cup honey or maple syrup
- 1/4 cup almond butter
- 1 teaspoon vanilla extract

Instructions:

1. Preheat oven to 350°F (175°C).

2. In a bowl, combine rolled oats, chopped almonds, shredded coconut, honey or maple syrup, almond butter, and vanilla extract.
3. Mix until well combined.
4. Press mixture into a lined baking dish.
5. Bake for 20-25 minutes, until golden brown.
6. Let cool completely before cutting into bars.

Nutritional Information (per bar):
- Calories: 180
- Protein: 5g
- Fat: 10g
- Carbohydrates: 20g
- Fiber: 3g

15. Frozen Banana Bites

Ingredients:
- 2 bananas, peeled and cut into bite-sized pieces
- 1/4 cup almond butter
- 1/4 cup dark chocolate chips

Instructions:
1. Line a baking sheet with parchment paper.
2. Spread almond butter onto banana pieces.
3. Place banana pieces on the prepared baking sheet.
4. Melt dark chocolate chips in the microwave or over a double boiler.
5. Drizzle melted chocolate over banana pieces.
6. Freeze for 2 hours, or until chocolate is set.
7. Serve frozen.

Nutritional Information:
- Calories: 160
- Protein: 3g
- Fat: 9g
- Carbohydrates: 20g
- Fiber: 4g

16. Pumpkin Pie Energy Balls

Ingredients:
- 1 cup rolled oats
- 1/2 cup canned pumpkin puree
- 1/4 cup almond butter
- 1/4 cup maple syrup
- 1 teaspoon pumpkin pie spice
- 1/4 cup chopped pecans

Instructions:
1. In a bowl, combine rolled oats, pumpkin puree, almond butter, maple syrup, pumpkin pie spice, and chopped pecans.
2. Mix until well combined.
3. Roll into bite-sized balls using your hands.
4. Refrigerate for at least 30 minutes before serving.

Nutritional Information (per ball):
- Calories: 100
- Protein: 3g
- Fat: 5g
- Carbohydrates: 12g
- Fiber: 2g

17. Chocolate Avocado Truffles

Ingredients:
- 2 ripe avocados
- 1/4 cup cocoa powder
- 1/4 cup honey or maple syrup
- 1 teaspoon vanilla extract
- Shredded coconut or cocoa powder for rolling

Instructions:
1. Scoop avocado flesh into a blender or food processor.
2. Add cocoa powder, honey or maple syrup, and vanilla extract.
3. Blend until smooth and creamy.
4. Chill in the refrigerator for at least 30 minutes.
5. Roll into small balls and coat with shredded coconut or cocoa powder.
6. Serve chilled.

Nutritional Information (per truffle):
- Calories: 90
- Protein: 1g
- Fat: 5g
- Carbohydrates: 12g
- Fiber: 3g

18. Sweet Potato Toast with Almond Butter and Banana

Ingredients:
- 1 large sweet potato, cut into 1/2-inch slices
- 1/4 cup almond butter
- 1 banana, sliced
- Honey or maple syrup (optional)
- Cinnamon (optional)

Instructions:
1. Toast sweet potato slices in a toaster or toaster oven until tender.
2. Spread almond butter onto toasted sweet potato slices.
3. Top with banana slices.
4. Drizzle with honey or maple syrup and sprinkle with cinnamon if desired.
5. Serve immediately.

Nutritional Information:
- Calories: 220
- Protein: 5g
- Fat: 10g
- Carbohydrates: 30g
- Fiber: 6g

19. Mango Lime Sorbet

Ingredients:
- 2 cups frozen mango chunks
- 1/4 cup lime juice
- 1/4 cup honey or maple syrup
- Fresh mint leaves for garnish (optional)

Instructions:
1. In a blender, combine frozen mango chunks, lime juice, and honey or maple syrup.
2. Blend until smooth.
3. Transfer mixture to a shallow dish and freeze for 2-3 hours, stirring occasionally.
4. Serve scoops of sorbet garnished with fresh mint leaves if desired.

Nutritional Information (per serving):
- Calories: 140
- Protein: 1g
- Fat: 0.5g
- Carbohydrates: 36g
- Fiber: 3g

20. Almond Flour Banana Bread

Ingredients:

- 2 cups almond flour
- 1 teaspoon baking soda
- 1/2 teaspoon salt
- 1 teaspoon ground cinnamon
- 3 ripe bananas, mashed
- 1/4 cup honey or maple syrup
- 1/4 cup coconut oil, melted
- 3 eggs
- 1 teaspoon vanilla extract

Instructions:

1. Preheat oven to 350°F (175°C). Grease a loaf pan or line with parchment paper.
2. In a bowl, combine almond flour, baking soda, salt, and ground cinnamon.
3. In another bowl, mash bananas and stir in honey or maple syrup, melted coconut oil, eggs, and vanilla extract.
4. Mix wet ingredients into dry ingredients until well combined.
5. Pour batter into prepared loaf pan.
6. Bake for 50-60 minutes, until a toothpick inserted into the center comes out clean.
7. Let cool in the pan for 10 minutes before transferring to a wire rack to cool completely.

Nutritional Information (per slice, based on 12 slices):
- Calories: 220   - Protein: 6g   - Fat: 15g
- Carbohydrates: 18g   - Fiber: 3g

CHAPTER 6: IMPORTANT ADVICE FOR TREATING HASHIMOTO'S THYROIDITIS

There is more to managing Hashimoto's thyroiditis than just dietary changes. It calls for a comprehensive strategy that includes recognizing your body's signals, managing stress, and making lifestyle adjustments. This chapter offers vital advice and strategies to support you in overcoming the obstacles of having Hashimoto's disease and achieving optimal health.

Comprehending Hashimoto's Thyroiditis

An autoimmune disorder called Hashimoto's thyroiditis causes the thyroid gland to be attacked by the immune system, which can cause inflammation and eventual damage over time. The thyroid gland may become hypothyroid as a result, producing insufficient hormones to meet the body's demands. Fatigue, weight gain, cold sensitivity, and dry skin are typical symptoms.

1. Cooperate closely with your medical staff

An endocrinologist and your physician make up part of your healthcare team, which is essential to managing Hashimoto's thyroiditis. To check thyroid hormone levels and make any prescription adjustments, routine check-ups and blood tests are crucial. Together with your medical professionals, create a customized treatment plan that takes into account your unique requirements.

2. Adhere to Your Suggested Treatment Schedule

Follow your doctor's instructions if you've been prescribed thyroid hormone replacement therapy (such as levothyroxine). Regular use of medicine helps reduce the symptoms of hypothyroidism and stabilize thyroid hormone levels. It's crucial to avoid changing your prescription dosage without first speaking with your doctor.

3. Make a Diet Rich in Nutrients

Thyroid function and general health can be enhanced by eating a diet high in nutrients. Prioritize entire meals that are high in antioxidants, vitamins, and minerals. Make sure your meals are rich in fruits, veggies, lean proteins, and healthy fats. Processed food items, refined sugars, and excessive caffeine should be minimized or avoided as they might have an adverse effect on thyroid health.

4. Track Iodine Consumption

The synthesis of thyroid hormones depends on iodine, but too much or too little of it might interfere with thyroid function. Make sure you are getting the right quantity of iodine in your diet, particularly if you are deficient or over-consuming it. Common dietary sources of iodine include seafood, dairy products, and iodized salt.

5. Effectively Handle Stress

Stress can impact general health and worsen the symptoms of Hashimoto's thyroiditis. Use stress-reduction strategies including yoga, meditation, deep breathing, and frequent exercise. Discover ways to de-stress and rejuvenate yourself, since this will enhance your overall health and lessen the negative effects of stress on your immune system.

6. Give Good Sleep First Priority

Immune system performance, hormone balance, and general health all depend on getting enough sleep. Aim for seven to nine hours of sleep every night, and create a calming evening ritual. Maintaining a cold, calm, and dark bedroom will help you fall asleep. To encourage sound sleep, avoid engaging in stimulating activities or using screens just before bed.

7. Get Regular Exercise

Frequent exercise promotes overall health, metabolism, and thyroid function. As advised by health guidelines, partake in moderate aerobic exercises like swimming, cycling, or walking for a minimum of 150 minutes per week. Exercises that focus on strength training can also support a healthy metabolism and help preserve muscle mass.

8. Pay Attention to Your Body

Pay heed to your body's signals and symptoms. Every day, record your feelings and take notice of any shifts or patterns. By being aware of these things, you can find circumstances that aggravate or cause your Hashimoto's thyroiditis. Share any worries or changes in your health with your healthcare staff in an open and honest manner.

9. Learn About Hashimoto's Disease

Knowing the fundamental causes of Hashimoto's thyroiditis will enable you to make wise decisions regarding your well-being. Keep up with the latest findings, available therapies, and recommended lifestyle changes for the management of autoimmune diseases. To access more resources and help, look for trustworthy information sources and think about joining online forums or support groups.

10. Take Up Your Health Cause

Engage in proactive health management and demand attention for your needs. Take the initiative to make routine check-ups, ask questions at doctor's appointments, and talk with your healthcare provider about available treatments. To get the best possible health results, work together with your healthcare team and maintain open lines of communication.

You may improve your general health and effectively manage Hashimoto's thyroiditis by putting these techniques and tips into practice. Keep in mind that every person's experience with Hashimoto's is different, so it could take some trial and error to figure out what suits you the best over time. Adopt a holistic approach to health that places an emphasis on taking care of yourself, making educated decisions, and having a positive outlook on managing your illness.

CONCLUSION

Living with Hashimoto's thyroiditis brings difficulties, but it also presents chances for development, fortitude, and a better comprehension of our own bodies. You have learned about the complexities of controlling this autoimmune disease during this trip, covering everything from dietary modifications to lifestyle adjustments and all in between. As our investigation comes to an end, it's critical to consider what we've discovered and how you can proceed with self-assurance and empowerment.

Understanding is the first step towards managing Hashimoto's thyroiditis. You have studied the basics of this illness and understand how autoimmune reactions can impact thyroid function and general health. Equipped with this knowledge, you've adopted a diet high in nutrients, realizing the benefits of whole foods for inflammation reduction and thyroid health support. You now understand the significance of iodine balance, how stress affects symptoms, how to integrate stress-reduction strategies, and how to prioritize restful sleep and regular exercise in order to promote resilience and vigor.

Finding balance is an ongoing effort that calls both perseverance and patience. You've learned that it's important to pay attention to your body and to take care of it by eating healthily, getting enough sleep, and engaging in activities that suits your needs. You've adjusted your treatment plan in close collaboration with your medical team, guaranteeing ideal thyroid hormone levels and effective symptom control. You now feel more capable of advocating for your health and maintaining control over your overall well-being thanks to this collaborative approach.

Holistic health includes mental and emotional well-being in addition to physical health. You've adopted mindfulness techniques, developing resilience in the face of adversity and an optimistic outlook. You have learned about triggers and patterns through education and self-awareness, which has empowered proactive symptom control. Your excellent support system and emphasis on self-care have fostered holistic health, which is the cornerstone for living well with Hashimoto's thyroiditis.

Recall that controlling Hashimoto's thyroiditis is a journey rather than a destination as you look to the future. With the information and resources at your disposal to handle life's ups and downs, greet each day with optimism and fortitude. Maintain your education by keeping up with developments in lifestyle and treatment approaches. Participate in support groups and get power from people's common experiences and viewpoints.

To sum up, the key to managing Hashimoto's thyroiditis is to identify your own route to wellness, which will be influenced by your commitment to living a healthy lifestyle, self-discovery, and perseverance. Honor your accomplishments, no matter how modest, and recognize the strides you've made in the process. Have faith in your capacity to overcome obstacles and grow and adapt. Recall that your perseverance and strength are what define you every day, not your illness.

As we come to the end of our discussion on how to manage thyroiditis caused by Hashimoto's, I want to encourage you to face your journey with bravery and compassion. Every step you take toward wellbeing is evidence of your power, and your health and well-being are worth nurturing. Empowered by knowledge, resilience, and optimism, you have the basis to lead a lively and fulfilling life with a supportive community by your side.

Together, let's go forward in our pursuit of wellbeing and self-determination despite having Hashimoto's thyroiditis. We can create a future where people with autoimmune illnesses thrive by campaigning for increased awareness, supporting one another, and sharing our stories. Your experience is special, worthwhile, and deserves recognition. May you always greet each day with grace and determination, understanding that you are not walking this road to well-being alone.

Finally, I would like to express my sincere wishes for your continuing health and wellbeing. May your path be one of strength, your decisions bring you comfort, and your capacity to fully experience life give you empowerment. May you confidently and optimistically manage the difficulties of Hashimoto's thyroiditis with information as your guide and resilience as your ally. Cheers to a future full of health, energy, and all the opportunities that lie ahead of you.